Table of content

Introduction

Chapter 1

Chapter 2

Chapter 3

Chapter 4

Chapter 5

Chapter 6

Conclusion

Introduction

Your Step-by-Step Guide on How to Extract Snail Mucin

The Secret to Youthful Skin: Unleashing the Power of Snail Mucin for Profit and Beauty"

The Sparkling Goo: Guide to Ethical Snail Mucus Extraction Forget diamonds, snail mucus is the real treasure! This sparkling secretion has been coveted for centuries for its legendary skin-transforming abilities. But have you ever wondered: what exactly is this magical substance and how can you get your hands on it ethically (without harming a sleazy friend)?

This book is your roadmap to the world of snail mucus. We'll reveal the secrets of this powerful elixir as we explore it: Glow power: Discover the science behind the impressive benefits of snail mucin, from moisturising and reducing wrinkles to fade scars and even have the ability to fight acne. Sustainable Slimming:

Learn how to extract snail mucus ethically, ensuring the health of our stomach friends and minimising environmental impact. No forced slime here! DIY Delight: Discover the secret to extracting your own snail mucus at home, with step-by-step instructions for soaking, boiling, and even fermenting (for the truly adventurous). Beyond the Face:

Expand your snail-energising horizons with recipes for hair rinses, soothing body baths, and even homemade snail mucus sheet masks! Forget harsh chemicals and questionable beauty standards. This book lets you harness the natural sheen of snail mucus while respecting both nature and our slimy little friends. So, open the book, unleash your inner alchemist and prepare to experience the transformative power of ethical snail slime!

Chapter 1

A. Mucin Magic goodness Snail mucus, those sparkly trails of slime you leave behind when you're... well, a snail, has unexpectedly found its way to our vanities. Stop frowning! Listen to me. This slimy elixir has some potential benefits that may make you reconsider your distaste. Imagine a tiny snail gliding across dew-drenched grass, its shimmering trail not only a trail marker but also a potent cocktail of skin-nourishing ingredients. Of course, snail mucus, harvested legally,

contains large amounts of: Moisturising power: Hyaluronic Acid, a natural hydration magnet, is boosted from snail mucus , helps your skin become plump and moisturised. Wrinkle Warrior: Antioxidants and collagen-boosting products help smooth out wrinkles and firm your skin. Soothes burns: Anti-inflammatory properties soothe irritated skin, becoming a close friend to sensitive and acne-prone souls.

Reduces Scars: This sticky goo can help reduce the appearance of acne scars and other stubborn scars. It's like a little snail carrying a personal care kit, ready to share its magic! Curious? Although research is still underway, snail mucus may be worth a try for your skin testing is essential and ethical sourcing is a must. So drop your scepticism and embrace the magic of mucus – your skin will probably thank you!

B. Don't Nap with Snails: The Importance of Ethical Mucus Extraction Snail Mucus, the Skin Care World's Latest Favourite, Carries the Weight of Expectations About Small Snails. Although it promises to work wonders on your skin, the extraction process should not leave behind any ethical concerns.

Here's why extracting snail mucus is important: Snail Health: Imagine small snails, stressed and injured, producing below average levels of mucus jar. It's disgusting! Ethical harvesting prioritises snail welfare, using methods such as misting or gentle stimulation to encourage natural slime production.

It may take longer, but happy snails will make happy (and productive) mucus. Purity Matters: Imagine this: contaminated mucus is wreaking havoc on your skin. Not the shine you expected! Proper extraction includes sanitation, filtration, and a controlled environment to keep the mucus clean and potent. Think of it as a day at the snail spa, making sure the final product suits your face. Snail Durability: Remember that snails are partial

Chapter 2

Unravelling the snail's secret potion:
A. glimpse into the magical world of slime. Have you ever looked at a snail and thought, "That slime could be the key for eternal youth?" Oh, you're not alone! Snail mucus, the slimy trail left behind by our shelled friends, is making waves in the world of skin care, but before you get covered in slime, let's dive into the attraction of this slippery feeling.

Picture this: a tiny snail glides across a dewy meadow, leaving not just a trail but a potent cocktail of nature's best products. Of course, snail mucus, ethically harvested, is a treasure trove of skin-loving ingredients, like: Hydration Heroes: Hyaluronic Acid, a natural magnet for hydration, enhanced by snail mucus, leaving your skin feeling well-hydrated. garden.

Wrinkle Warrior: Antioxidants and collagen boosters work together to fight wrinkles and firm your skin, leaving you looking as youthful as a newly sprouted seedling. Soothes stings: Its anti-inflammatory properties soothe irritated skin, making it a friend to even the most sensitive souls. Think of it as a soothing balm for stressed skin.

Scar Fade Fighter: This fine oil can help reduce the appearance of acne scars and other stubborn marks, leaving your skin smoother than its freshly polished finish. But wait, there's more! Understanding snail mucus goes beyond its benefits. We must think of the little architects behind this wonderful elixir.

Ethical mining is essential, ensuring the well-being of our snail friends. Imagine a gentle mist or stimulation, encouraging them to safely share their drool. Think of it as a spa day for snails, with the added benefit of glowing skin for you as Research on snail mucus is still ongoing but its potential is undeniable.

So if you're curious about this unique ingredient, do your research, choose ethically sourced products and maybe, just maybe, you'll find that little magic bottle powered by Your own snail! Remember, don't expect immediate transformation.

Patience, like a snail navigating its path, is the key. And who knows, you might even develop a new fondness for our sleazy friends, those little alchemists who leave behind a trail of beauty secrets.
A Mystery revealed: What really is snail mucus? Forget magical potions and mythical beasts, the latest healing rumours come straight from the garden... slip on it, to be exact.

Yes, we're talking about snail mucus, the slimy trail left behind by these humble mollusks. But before you imagine yourself covered in slime, let's dive into the fascinating world of this natural wonder. Imagine a snail gliding gracefully across a dew-drenched leaf, leaving behind not just a trail of sparkle but also a powerful blend of nature's best skin care ingredients.

That's Snail Mucin: , a complex blend of proteins, hyaluronic acid, antioxidants and other goodies secreted by snails to keep their delicate bodies protected, hydrated and developed. Think of it as your snail's personal first aid kit, containing: Hydrate Hero: Hyaluronic acid, a natural hydration magnet, enhanced by snail mucus, helps skin Yours is like a well-watered garden.

Wrinkle Warrior: Antioxidants and collagen-boosting peptides work together to fight wrinkles and firm your skin, leaving you looking as youthful as a spring leaf. Soothes stings: Its anti-inflammatory properties soothe irritated skin, making snail mucus a friend to even the most sensitive souls. Think of it as a soothing balm for stressed skin.

Scar Fade Fighter: This sticky goo can help reduce the appearance of acne scars and other stubborn marks, leaving your skin smoother than a shiny seashell. But wait, snail explorers! Understanding snail mucus goes beyond its benefits.

We must consider the ethics of exploiting it. Imagine a gentle mist or stimulation, encouraging these little architects to safely share their drool. Think of it as a spa day for snails, with the added benefit of glowing skin for you!

Research into snail mucus continues but its potential is undeniable. So if you're curious about this unique ingredient, do your research, choose ethically sourced products and maybe, just maybe, you'll find your snail-powered magic bottle. only me.

Remember that patience is the key, like a snail finding its way. And who knows, you might even develop a new fondness for our sleazy friends, those little alchemists who leave behind a trail of beauty secrets.

B.Unravelling the snail's secret sauce: Delving into Gooey goodness Slip away, Cinderella's Carriage! The latest beauty rumour involves another type of cart, powered by slime: , the tiny snail. Forget the fairy tale transformation, let's dissect the reality of what makes these bloated gastropods glow: their own "snail mucus." Picture this: a tiny snail that not only leaves a trail of glitter but also releases a powerful elixir with each swipe.

This mucilage, ethically harvested, is a treasure trove of ingredients that can transform your skin care routine. But before we dive into the slime, let's explore its composition and properties: Mucus Inside: Hydration Hero: Hyaluronic acid, nature's hydration magnet, is boosted Enriched with snail mucus, it leaves your skin dewy. meadow after summer rain.

Wrinkle Warrior: antioxidants and collagen-boosting peptides work together to fight wrinkles and firm your skin, leaving you looking as youthful as a newly sprouted leaf.

Soothes stings: Anti-inflammatory properties soothe irritated skin, acting like a soothing balm for stressed skin, bringing relief to even the most sensitive souls. Scar Fade Fighter: This fine oil can help reduce the appearance of acne scars and other stubborn marks, leaving your skin smoother than its shiny finish.

Beyond the Goo: But understanding snail mucus goes beyond its benefits. We need to think about the happiness of our unkempt friends. Ethical harvesting is important as it ensures the process is like a spa day for the snails, encouraging them to share their slime safely. Imagine a gentle mist or stimulation, a far cry from the harshness of a fairy godmother's wand.

Disclosure: Research into snail mucus is still ongoing, but its potential is undeniable. So if you're curious about this unique ingredient, do your research, choose ethically sourced products and maybe, just maybe, you'll unlock the snail-powered magic pot's own slug.

Remember that patience is the key, like a snail finding its way. And who knows, you might even develop a new appreciation for these fascinating creatures, these little alchemists who leave a trail of beauty secrets. This is a transformation worth adopting!

C.Unexpected Snail Slime: Reveals Your Face's Goodness Moves, Serums, and Pills, There's a New Player in the Skin Care Game, and It's Slime, Shiny, and Effective surprising result: snail mucus. Stop frowning! Listen to me. This sticky elixir, left behind by our gardening friends, could be the key to regaining bright, youthful skin.

Imagine a snail that not only marks its territory but also creates a powerful mixture of nature's best products. Of course, Snail Mucus, ethically sourced, has many benefits: Hydration Hero: Forget about dry patches! Hyaluronic acid, a natural moisture magnet, is enhanced by snail mucus, leaving your skin like a well-hydrated oasis.

Wrinkle Warrior: Time goes back? Most of them! Antioxidants and collagen-boosting peptides work together to fight wrinkles and firm your skin, leaving you looking as youthful as a newly sprouted leaf. Soothe the sting: Redness and irritation? Go! The anti-inflammatory properties soothe your skin, acting as a soothing balm for even the most sensitive souls.

Scar Fade Fighter: The stubborn mark is hiding? Snail mucus could be your secret weapon. This fine oil can help reduce the appearance of acne scars and other blemishes, leaving your skin smoother than a shiny seashell. But wait, there's more to tell! Ethical mining is key. Imagine these little architects, uninjured, but encouraged to share their saliva through misting or gentle stimulation.

Think of it as a spa day with snails, with the added benefit of glowing skin for you! Snail secretion process before processing: Remember, research on snail mucus is still ongoing but its potential is undeniable. So, before using slime, do your research and choose products from legal sources. Who knows, you might find your own snail-powered magic jar!

Remember that patience is the key, like a snail moving slowly on its way. And who knows, you might even develop a new appreciation for these fascinating creatures, these little alchemists who leave a trail of beauty secrets. This is a respectable transformation, slime and all!

Chapter 3

From Snail Tracks to Skin Care Warehouse: Navigating Ethical Mucin Snail Mucin, the Slimy Pioneer of the Skin Care World, Has Potential Benefits From Moisturizing to Reducing wrinkle. But before we embark on the snail race, let's delve into the murky waters to source this fascinating ingredient. Imagine a snail that not only leaves a sparkling trail but also releases a powerful elixir with each swipe.

This mucilage is harvested ethically and is key to unleashing its potential. But ethical sourcing is not a fairy tale: it requires conscious choices. Avoid slimy bellies: Be careful with salt mines: Forget harsh methods like salt baths, which stress and harm snails. Look for brands that favour gentle extractions, like misting or stimulation, similar to a luxurious snail spa day.

Happy Snails, Happy Skin: Prioritise closed systems where snails thrive in natural environments, not factory farms. Think happy snails, healthy mucus and happier skin! Transparency is key: looks for brands that publicly share their sourcing and certification practices with organisations like Leaping Bunny, ensuring ethical and tamper-free processing cruelty.

Beyond ethics: Remember, research on snail mucus is still ongoing. While the potential is enticing, consider doing a patch test before diving headfirst into the slime. Choose ethically sourced products that align with your values and embrace a journey of discovery.

From Garden Glide to Glowing Skin: By understanding the importance of ethical sourcing, you can navigate the mucus maze and make informed choices. Who knows, you might unlock a magical bottle of snail power, not just for your skin but for the health of these fascinating creatures.

And who doesn't want that kind of transforming light? So be curious, ask questions and choose wisely. After all, beauty should not be at the expense of the happiness of others. Now that's a story worth telling! A Snail Spa or Slime Slam? Mucin Mania Ethical Disclosure Snail mucin, a pioneer in skin care, is touted for its moisturising, wrinkle-reducing and soothing properties.

But before you sink your teeth into this creamy goodness, let's demystify the mysteries of sourcing this trendy ingredient. Imagine a snail that not only leaves a trail of glitter but also brews a powerful elixir with each swipe. This mucus, ethically sourced, will of course unleash its true potential. But ethical sourcing is no fairy tale; it requires thoughtful choices. Avoid slime mines: Avoid salt mines: Forget about harsh methods like salt baths that stress and harm snails.

Look for brands that prioritise gentle extractions, such as misting or stimulation. Think of it as a luxury spa day for snails, not a brutal mining site. Happy Snails, Happy Skin: Closed systems where snails thrive in natural environments and not industrial farms are essential. Imagine happy snails, healthy mucus, and light-reflecting skin inside there! Transparency is key: Look for brands that publicly share their sourcing and certification practices with organisations like Leaping Bunny.

Their reaction will make your skin glow with confidence, not discomfort. Beyond ethics: Remember, research on snail mucus is still ongoing. While the potential is enticing, you should patch test before diving headfirst into the slime. Choose ethically sourced products that align with your values and embark on a journey of informed discovery.

From Garden Glide to Glowing Conscience: By understanding the importance of ethical sourcing, you can navigate the slime maze and make informed choices. Who knows, you might unlock a magical bottle of snail power, not just for your skin but for the health of these fascinating creatures. And who doesn't want that kind of transforming light? So be curious, ask questions and choose wisely. After all,
beauty should not be at the expense of the happiness of others. Now that's a story worth telling!

A. Snail Spa or Slime Slam? Mucin Mania Ethical Disclosure Snail mucin, a pioneer in skin care, is touted for its moisturising, wrinkle-reducing and soothing properties. But before you sink your teeth into this creamy goodness, let's demystify the mysteries of sourcing this trendy ingredient.

Imagine a snail that not only leaves a trail of glitter but also brews a powerful elixir with each swipe. This mucus, ethically sourced, will of course unleash its true potential. But ethical sourcing is no fairy tale; it requires thoughtful choices. Avoid slime mines:

Avoid salt mines: Forget about harsh methods like salt baths that stress and harm snails. Look for brands that prioritise gentle extractions, such as misting or stimulation. Think of it as a luxury spa day for snails, not a brutal mining site. Happy

Snails, Happy Skin: Closed systems where snails thrive in natural environments and not industrial farms are essential. Imagine happy snails, healthy mucus, and light-reflecting skin inside there! Transparency is key: Look for brands that publicly share their sourcing and certification practices with organisations. Don't hesitate to ask questions; Their reaction will make your skin glow with confidence, not discomfort.

Beyond ethics: Remember, research on snail mucus is still ongoing. While the potential is enticing, you should patch test before diving headfirst into the slime. Choose ethically sourced products that align with your values and embark on a journey of informed discovery.

From Garden Glide to Glowing Conscience: By understanding the importance of ethical sourcing, you can navigate the slime maze and make informed choices. Who knows, you might unlock a magical bottle of snail power, not just for your skin but for the health of these fascinating creatures.

And who doesn't want that kind of transforming light? So be curious, ask questions and choose wisely. After all, beauty should not be at the expense of the happiness of others. This is a story worth telling, one in which you and the snails can truly shine!

B. Selectivity: Choosing the right gastropod for snail slime goodness Snail mucus, the skin care world's newest favourite, might make you wonder: Are all traces of snail slime created equal? Buckle up, beauty adventurers, because choosing the right gastropod for mucus extraction doesn't have to be a chore!

Imagine a lively snail selection process, based not on speed or shell size but on ethical considerations and the magic of mucus. Let's ditch our slimy shrouds and explore inside an ethical snail sanctuary: Species spotlight: Leave the garden gnomes alone: Common encounters with wild snails with stress and danger.

Look for brands that work with farm-raised species like Helix Aspera Müller, ensuring their health throughout their mucus-making journey. Diversity matters: Forget monocultures! Look for brands that support biodiversity by using a variety of snail species, enriching ecosystems and promoting responsible agricultural practices.

Beyond the Shell: Snail Spa, Not Slug Slog: Ditch harsh extraction methods like salt baths. Choose brands that favour gentle stimulation or misting techniques, giving your snail a relaxing spa experience (with the added benefit of quality mucus!). Happy snails, healthy mucus: Closed system is the key!

Look for brands that provide a natural, stress-free environment for snails, promoting optimal health and, therefore, superior mucus quality. Celebrate Certifications: Leaping Bunny is Your Best Friend: Choose brands with certifications from organisations like Leaping Bunny, which ensure cruelty-free practices and the ethical treatment of people our sleazy friend. Remember, beauty has a conscience:

Research on snail mucus is ongoing, so approach with curiosity and caution. You should test the patch before applying the lubricant. But by choosing ethically sourced brands, you're not only investing in your skin, but also supporting sustainable practices and contributing to the well-being of these fascinating creatures.

So abandon your fairy godmother's magic wand and choose snail beauty with a clear conscience. After all, a glowing skin that celebrates ethical choices will outshine any diamond crown! Have fun tasting snails!

C. Snail-coal Sustainability: From Slime Stains to Eco-Friendly Scales Snail Mucus, Skin Care World's Slime Sensation, You May Be Wondering: Does Snail Farming Have Canned Be sustainable? Buckle up, eco-conscious explorers, because raising healthy, happy snails is about more than just beautiful skin:

It's about taking care of the planet! Imagine a snail farm that not only produces mucus but also grows in harmony with the environment. Let's ditch the sleazy stereotypes and dive into the world of sustainable snail education: Nature's playground:

Monoculture ditches: Forget rows of identical snail cages. Promote biodiversity by mimicking natural ecosystems, planting diverse vegetation and encouraging beneficial insects to control pests. Think of it as a Shangri-La snail! Don't waste, don't want:

Snail manure is not only waste but also nutrient-rich fertiliser for your farm! Opt for closed-loop systems that recycle waste back into the ground, creating a self-sufficient paradise. Water Wise: Conserve precious water resources by using efficient irrigation and rainwater harvesting systems. Every drop counts when it comes to snail sustainability!

Happy Snails, Happy Planet: Snail Spa, Stress Free Factory: Say no to harsh chemicals and cramped conditions. Choose humane measures such as natural light, spacious housing, and stress-free mucus collection. Imagine satisfied snails, producing peak mucus! Predators are partners:

Don't fight nature, join it! Encouraging natural predators like birds and frogs keeps insect populations in check, creating a balanced ecosystem where everyone thrives. Local is Snail-cial: Supports small, local snail farms that prioritise ethical practices and reduce emissions from transportation.

Think of it as reducing a snail's footprint! Remember that sustainability takes time: Research on snail mucus is ongoing, so take a long-term view. Choose brands that prioritise sustainable practices, even if it means waiting a little longer for your skin care solution. Every choice counts!

By adopting sustainable snail farming, you not only get ethically sourced mucus, but you also contribute to a healthier planet and happier snails. And who doesn't want that kind of shine? So, give up miracle solutions and choose snail beauty with a clear conscience. After all, a sustainable future is one in which both humans and snails can shine!

Chapter 4

A Secrets Revealed: Demystifying the Soothing Art of Mucin Magic Snail mucus, the skin care world's new favourite, makes us crave dewy skin and youthful fun. But before you use the slime, let's take a look behind the curtain of the extraction process - because ethical sourcing is as important as the final glow. Imagine a snail that not only leaves a trail of sparkles but also delivers a powerful elixir with every swipe.

Snail mucus, harvested legally, is of course the key to unleashing its true potential. But ditch the harsh chemical baths and salt mines often involved in mucus extraction - we're talking snail spa days, not slimy torture chambers! Gentle Stimulation, Big Reward: Consider a Gentle Mist:

Imagine snails happily enjoying a refreshing shower of water, enticing them to share their healthy mucus naturally. It's like a spa treatment, without the cucumbers (they prefer lettuce anyway). Purposeful stimulation: Gentle petting or brushing can help, encouraging them to release their precious mucus without any stress or harm.

Think of it as a friendly game of fetch, with mucus as a reward. Mimic Nature's Generosity: Some farms even use natural stimuli such as plants or specific scents, tapping into the innate behaviours of these fascinating creatures. It's like speaking their unforgettable language, promoting trust and cooperation. From Snails to Hideouts:

Fine Slime Purification: Natural Filtration System: After gentle collection, the mucus can be filtered through natural materials such as activated carbon, removing impurities while retaining its delicate properties. Think of it as a natural spa treatment for mucus itself. Celebrating Centrifugation : Imagine a gentle spinning cycle, separating pure mucus from any remaining particles.

It's like a snail-approved washing machine, ensuring impeccable quality without the use of harsh chemicals. Freeze-drying magic: Want to preserve the power of mucus? Look for brands that use freeze-drying techniques, which retain all the good stuff without compromising their effectiveness.

Think of it as a cryo-sleep for the mucus, ensuring it stays fresh and potent. Remember, patience is key: Unlike the instant fairy tales, research on snail mucus is still ongoing. You should patch the test before diving headfirst into slime.

Choose ethically sourced brands that align with your values and embark on an informed journey of discovery. So ditch the harsh extraction methods and choose snail beauty to respect both you and these fascinating creatures. After all, glowing skin based on ethical choices will shine brighter than any diamond crown! Have fun tasting snails!

B .Snail Management: From vile companions comes Maintainable Snail Slime, the skin care world's newest slimy sensation, making us imagine dewy skin and youthful happiness. But now that you've covered yourself in mud, let's dive into the world of snail collecting and care – because ethical treatment is the establishment of true excellence.

Imagine a field not only filled with snails but also bustling with respect and care. Collecting and managing snails, when done properly, can be a pleasant gesture between humans and these interesting animals. Throw away those cruel shovels and nets: we're talking snail havens, not vile stampede parties! Delicate, Sensitive Mammoths:

Happy Snails, Optimistic Goo: Imagine a quiet, calm environment where snails can thrive. Think light, spacious enclosed spaces and loads of leafy snacks – a snail's paradise! In fact, happy snails provide higher quality mucus. Carefully picked up by hand: Imagine gentle hands carefully picking up snails, avoiding being pushed and injured.

It is like picking a flower that is sensitive to the excellence and delicacy of life. Fresh & Collected: Remember that snails are very sensitive to temperature changes. Legitimate care includes cool situations and delicate movements, ensuring their health throughout the process. The Enchantment of Slime, Ethical Source:

Less is More: Don't Collect Too Much! The maintainable tools consist of collecting, so to speak, a small patch of snail mucus, allowing them to regenerate and grow. Think of it as sharing, not taking everything away. Hydration Hero: Once collected, give the snail a revitalising mist or go to a place with clean water.

It's like a post-spa treatment, ensuring they stay upbeat and hydrated. Discharge and Celebrate: Once the mucus is collected, carefully return the snails to their typical living space. It's like giving them a ticket back home, ensuring a cycle of support. Remember that snail beauty takes time:

Research on snail mucus is ongoing, so take a long-term view. Choose brands that prioritise ethical sourcing and treatment, even if it means you have to wait a little longer to get your skin care fix. Every choice is verified! By holding an Ethical Snail Collection and caring for it, you are not only receiving ethically sourced mucus, but you are also contributing to a world where humans and snails can live in harmony .

And who wouldn't need that shine? So, skip the quick solutions and choose the excellence delivered by snail with all your heart. After all, an achievable future is one in which both men and snails can shine!

B. Snail spa day: Removes greasy mucus (no burning pain) Snail mucus, the skin care world's newest sticky diamond, ensures hydration, fights wrinkles and gives some shine. But lately you've been diving headfirst into the alluvial layer, looking behind the shadow of mining.

Ethical sourcing is not a buzzword; it is the establishment of true excellence. Ignore the image of snails gathering under a chemical shower! Imagine a subtle, snail-centric approach: Subtle influences of nature: Moisturisers: Imagine happy snails receiving an invigorating dose of spray , often prompting them to share their mucus benefits.

Think of it as a spa treatment, without the cucumbers (they lean toward lettuce). Reminder with reason: Gentle petting or brushing can do the job, allowing them to release their precious contents without stretching or damage. Think of it as exciting entertainment, with mucus as a reward.

Natural Clues: Some farms use signature enhancements such as specific plants or scents, exploiting the natural behaviour of these interesting creatures. It's like speaking their vile language, fostering trust and engagement. From snail slime to skin care reserves: Nature's filter: Next gently collected, the mucus can be filtered through natural materials such as activated carbon, removing impurities while retaining its delicate properties.

Think of it as a natural spa treatment for mucus itself. Celebrating centrifugation: Imagine a gentle spinning cycle, separating pure mucus from any remaining particles. It's like a snail-approved washing machine, ensuring impeccable quality without the use of harsh chemicals.

Freeze-drying magic: Want to preserve the power of mucus? Look for brands that use freeze-drying techniques, which retain all the good stuff without compromising their effectiveness. Think of it as a cryo-sleep for the mucus, ensuring it stays fresh and potent. Remember, patience is key:

Research on snail mucus is ongoing, so it's a good idea to try the patch before diving headfirst into the slime. Choose ethically sourced brands that align with your values and embark on an informed journey of discovery as you ditch the harsh extraction methods and choose snail beauty that respects both you and these fascinating creatures. After all, glowing skin based on ethical choices will shine brighter than any diamond crown! Have fun tasting snails!

C. From Garden Glide to Glowing Skin: Purifies and Preserves the Magic of Snail Mucus The skin care world's newest slime, promising buds Smile hydrated, wrinkle-free.

But before you immerse yourself in the slime, let's delve into the hidden world of purification and preservation. Just like Cinderella needs more than a pumpkin, mucus needs a little magic to turn into skincare gold.

Picture this: a sparkling path, one that not only marks the snail's path but is also filled with potential. Ethical sourcing is key, so imagine gentle misting or playful stimulation, a far cry from brutal exploitation. Now the collected substance needs its own treatment process:

Natural treatments: Fiesta filter: Activated carbon acts like a friendly sponge, absorbing impurities while still maintaining good quality. Think of it as a natural detox, keeping mucus healthy and pure. Celebrating centrifugation:

Imagine a gentle spin, like a merry-go-round for microscopic particles. This separates pure mucus, ensuring optimal quality without the need for harsh chemicals. Think of it as a snail-approved washing machine!

Freeze-drying: Have you ever heard of freeze-drying for skin care? Freeze-drying locks in all the good stuff, like the well-timed pause button. This preserves the potency of the mucus, ensuring that it stays fresh and ready to work its magic.

But the journey doesn't end there: Natural preservatives: Forget harsh chemicals! Look for brands that use natural preservatives like rosemary extract or vitamin E. Think of it as a plant shield, protecting mucus from unwanted guests. Fresh & Collected:

Just as snails love dewy mornings, mucilage thrives in cool temperatures. Proper storage, like sleeping in the refrigerator, keeps him happy and energetic.

Fresh is best: Snail mucus is not like fine wine; It doesn't get better with age. Choose products with clear expiration dates and use within the recommended time frame. Think of it as respecting the purity of nature's goodness. Remember that beauty takes time: Research on snail mucus is still ongoing, so be patient.

You should check the patches before diving headfirst into the slime. Choose ethically sourced brands that prioritise purity and preservation, even if it means waiting a little longer for your skin care solution. Every choice counts!

By understanding the magic of purification and preservation, you not only achieve effective skin care but also support responsible practices and respect the little alchemists who leave their traces This shimmer. So embark on the journey, choose wisely and let your skin shine knowing that beauty and ethics can go hand in hand. After all, snail skin that shines with responsibility is truly the ending of a fairy tale!

Chapter 5

Snail Stories: Unleash Your Face's Good Mucus Snail mucus, the new crown jewel of the skin care world, promises hydrated, anti-wrinkle and glowing skin. But before we immerse ourselves in slime like a princess in a fairy tale, let's learn about the art of applying it. There are no pumpkin recipes here, just thoughtful techniques for harnessing the power of this unique ingredient.

A shimmering trail left by a little architect, not only marks its path but also holds the key to radiant skin. Ethical sourcing is paramount, so imagine a gentle mist or playful stimulation, not a harsh exploitation. Now the purified and preserved mucus is waiting to invade your face:

Snail Eating Ritual: Clean as a Gliding Snail: Imagine a clean and sparkling dew-covered meadow . Start with a gentle cleanser to remove impurities, creating a new base for the magical mucus. Remember, staying clean means better absorption!

Less is more, snail style: Don't go too far! A pea-sized amount of mucus is enough. Imagine a small snail leaving a mark, delicate and fragile. Apply evenly to the face and neck, avoiding the delicate eye area. Gentle touches, big results: Think gentle circular movements, mimicking the gentle sliding motion of a snail.

Massage the mucus into your skin and let it be absorbed like morning dew on a thirsty meadow. It can be done at breakneck speed, but the results can be transformative! Caution Type: Snail mucus mixed with other substances!

Wait until the mucus is completely absorbed before applying your regular moisturiser or serum. Think of it as building a harmonious ecosystem on your skin, with each layer complementing the next.

But remember that snail magic takes time: Test your skin before peeling: Not all skin likes all the ingredients. Do a patch test on the inside of your arm 24 hours before applying it all over your face. Consistency is key:

Just as a snail leaves its mark day after day, regular use is important. Be patient and give your skin time to feel the benefits of the mucus.

You won't change overnight, but if you persevere, you'll see radiant skin appear. Listen to your skin: Each skin is unique, like the tracks of each snail. Pay attention to how your skin reacts and adjust your routine accordingly. Sometimes less really is more! Embrace the spirit of the snail: Choosing ethically sourced snail mucus isn't just about your skin;

It's about respecting these fascinating creatures. So take a slow and steady approach, appreciate the natural world, and let your skin reflect not only your beauty but also your ethical choices. After all, the shining light of responsibility is truly a fairy tale ending – no magic wand needed!

A.Snail Magic: Weaves Mucin Into Your Skin Care Symphony Snail Mucin , the skin care world's newest slimy muse, promises hydration, anti-wrinkle and natural shine.
But before you make your own DIY slime mask (trust us, skip that one!), explore the art of incorporating this unique ingredient into your current routine. Think of it not as a fairy godmother's wand but as a delicate instrument in your personal beauty orchestra.

Picture this: a shimmering trail left by a little architect, not only marking his path but also holding the key to radiant skin. Ethical sourcing is paramount, so imagine a gentle mist or playful stimulation, not a harsh extract. Now, purified and preserved mucin awaits harmonious integration into your skin care routine:

Snail Symphonies: Mix Mucin with other ingredients: Hydrate Harmony: Take a look Mucin from snails like oboe, enriches your moisturiser with its water-holding capacity. Magic. Imagine dewy meadows and succulent, plump skin singing in perfect harmony.

Anti-wrinkle duo: Combines mucin with peptides or retinol for a powerful anti-aging chorus. Imagine the slender lines fading like morning dew, leaving behind a softer, more youthful tone. Sonata Sonata: Sensitive skin? Mix mucus with soothing ingredients such as aloe vera or centella . Imagine the discomfort disappearing like a discordant note being replaced by a gentle, soothing melody.

Brightening Shine: Combine mucin with vitamin C or niacinamide for radiant, glowing skin. Imagine dull skin disappearing like darkness at dawn, leaving your skin illuminated with a healthy glow. Remember that a symphony takes practice: Start slowly: Don't overwhelm your skin! Introduce mucus gradually, starting with a few drops mixed into your existing products.

Listen to your skin's rhythm and adjust accordingly. Experimentation is key: Like a composer exploring different musical instruments, try combining different mucins with other ingredients to find the perfect harmony for your skin care. Friend. There is no one-size-fits-all approach! Patch Test Before Encore:

Not everyone's skin likes every ingredient. Perform a patch test on your inner arm 24 hours before adding mucus to your routine. Be kind to your skin, star of the show! Embrace the spirit of the snail: Choosing ethically sourced snail mucus isn't just about your skin; it's about respecting these fascinating creatures. So celebrate the natural world, appreciate the science behind sebum, and let your skin reflect not only beauty but also ethical choices.

After all, the brilliant light in harmony with the melody of nature is truly a beautiful work to behold. Now go ahead and create your own unique skin care symphony, with snail mucin as the secret ingredient!

B. Warning: Using snail mucus at home is potentially risky and is not recommended. It's true that snail mucus has been gaining a foothold in the world of skin care, but before we make our own DIY slime masks, let's stop. Although the potential benefits of snail mucin are appealing, using it at home also poses significant risks. Giving up the DIY dream:

Sourcing ethically: Sourcing ethically produced snail mucus is crucial and without the right knowledge and connections then that is almost impossible. Self-harvesting can harm the snails and reduce the quality of the mucus.
Remember, happy snails mean happy skin! Contamination concerns: DIY extraction and preparation lack the controlled environment and sterilisation techniques used by professionals.

Bacteria and other contaminants can lurk in homemade mucus, leading to irritation, infection, or worse. Snail slime is not a miracle drug; This requires careful handling. Quality Control: Purifying and preserving mucus for safe use requires specialised equipment and expertise. DIY attempts can leave you with an ineffective or even harmful recipe. Snail slime requires a science lab, not a kitchen counter.

Unproven effectiveness: Although there has been research on snail mucus, it is still in its infancy. Do-it-yourself testing lacks the scientific rigour and testing necessary to ensure its effectiveness or safety. Trust the experts, not luck, when it comes to your skin. Celebrate sustainable alternatives: Support ethical brands:

Look for brands committed to responsible snail farming and harvesting practices. Invest in quality, knowing that your skin and snails are treated with respect. Consult a dermatologist: Ask an expert about your specific skin concerns and whether professional snail mucin products might be right for you . They can guide you toward safe and effective solutions. Use natural alternatives:

Explore other natural ingredients with proven benefits, like hyaluronic acid or aloe vera. Nature has a treasure trove of options to explore! Remember that beauty should not come at the expense of your health or the welfare of animals.

Leave snail slime to the experts and discover safer and more ethical alternatives for your skin care journey. Let your light come from wise choices, not risky DIY experiments.

C.Electrocute your skin: Unleash the full power of snail mucus Snail mucus, the skin care world's newest slimy muse, promises to moisturise, fight wrinkles and deliver skin so bright that it could surpass the firefly festival. But before you soak yourself in slime and call it a day, hold your horses (or snails, as the case may be). Maximising the benefits of this unique ingredient requires a little finesse, like coaxing a shy snail out of its shell.

A streak of light shimmering in the moonlight, not only marking the way but also holding the key to radiant skin. Ethical sourcing is paramount, so imagine a gentle mist or playful stimulation, not a harsh extract. Now the purified and preserved mucus awaits its journey to your face, but remember, the magic needs a little boost: Sharpen your senses from your shell: The moisture harmony:

Think of your skin like a thirsty grassland. Prepare it with toner or moisturising essence before applying mucin. This creates a moisture-wicking foundation that maximises absorption and plumps the skin. Fiesta Exfoliation: Like removing overgrown foliage, gentle exfoliation removes dead skin cells, allowing mucus to penetrate deeper and work its magic more effectively .

But be gentle, snails won't want their delicate home scratched! Subclass like snail architect: Snail slime works well with others! Follow up the mucus with your regular moisturiser and serum, creating a delicious layer cake. Think of it as building an ecosystem that protects and nourishes your skin. Snail Speed Patience:

Don't expect results overnight. Like the steady journey of a snail, regular use over time will bring out the full potential of mucus. Be patient, let the magic work its magic and enjoy the gradual transformation. Remember that the secret of snails is not a fairy tale: Patch test before peeling: Not all skin likes all ingredients. Perform a patch test on the inside of your arm 24 hours before applying the mucus to your entire face.

Listen to your skin, it is the conductor of your beauty symphony. Knowledgeable Storage: Snail mucus, like fresh produce, prefers cool, dark environments. Store in the refrigerator to preserve its potency and effectiveness. Don't let your snail magic fade! Ethical choices shine brightest:

Choosing responsibly sourced mucus isn't just about your skin, it's also about respecting these fascinating creatures. Support brands committed to ethical practices and let your halo reflect the good choices you make. Embracing the spirit of the snail: Harnessing the full potential of snail mucus is more than just using a product;

It's about respecting nature and appreciating the science behind good. So celebrate the natural world, make wise choices and let your skin radiate not only beauty but also ethical awareness. After all, shining with responsibility is truly attractive, and it's a beauty secret that even the most beautiful princess in a fairy tale can't afford. Now get out there, explore and let your skin sparkle with the power of a snail!

Chapter 6

Snail Investigation: Reveals the Safety Side of Mucin's Magic Snail Mucin, Skin Care World's Latest Glittery Guest, Promises Hydration, Wrinkle Reverse, and Bright Shine brighter than a firefly conference. But before you dive headfirst into this sleazy trend, let's put on our detective hats and investigate the safety side of things. Remember, responsible beauty will shine brighter than any diamond crown! Picture this: a shimmering path that not only marks the way but also holds the potential for radiant skin.

Ethical sourcing is key, so imagine a gentle mist or playful stimulation, not a harsh extract. Now the purified and preserved mucus awaits its journey to your face, but remember, safety first: Patch Test, Don't Guess: Not everyone's skin is your friend every ingredient. Perform a 24-hour patch test on the inside of your arm before applying the snail mask.

Think of it as a secret handshake; Your skin needs to be approved before you fully embrace it. Listen to your skin: Like a trusty snail, pay attention to your skin's signals. Redness, itching or irritation? Take a step back! Not all snail mucus is created equal and your skin may throw a little tantrum.

Consult Derma-Detective: Don't know if you should use snail slime? Consult a dermatologist, an expert in optimal skin care. They can evaluate your skin, answer your questions, and guide you toward safe and effective solutions. DIY?

Not today: Even though the internet whispers sweet things about homemade snail mucus, resist the urge! Sourcing ethically and ensuring good hygiene is difficult and the risks of contamination outweigh the potential benefits. Leave the science to the experts! Understanding Preservation:

Snail mucus is not a fairy medicine; he needs proper care. Store it in the refrigerator to preserve its potency and prevent growth from unwanted guests. Think of it as giving mucin a cool, refreshing spa experience. Ethical choices shine brightest: Choosing responsibly sourced mucus isn't just about your skin; it's about respecting these fascinating creatures.

Support brands committed to ethical practices and let your halo reflect the good choices you make. Remember, beauty with awareness truly shines! Embrace the spirit of the snail: Unlocking the potential of snail mucus is more than just using a product;

It's about appreciating science and respecting nature. So celebrate the natural world, make wise choices and let your skin radiate not only beauty but also ethical awareness. After all, shining with responsibility is truly captivating and it's a beauty secret that even the cunningest fairy tale villain can't steal. Now go out, explore responsibly, and let your skin shine with the power of wise choices!

A But be careful: Navigate the slimy side of Snail Mucin Snail Mucin, the new shimmery guest of the skincare world, promises youthful skin and anti-wrinkle magic . But before we dive into this slimy trend, let's peel back its glitter and consider the potential risks and allergies that may be lurking underneath. Remember, informed beauty always shines brighter than dreams!

A shimmering path leading to a dewy meadow, not only marking the path but also holding the potential for radiant skin. Ethical sourcing is paramount, so imagine a gentle mist or playful stimulation, not a harsh extract. Now the purified and preserved mucus awaits its journey to your face, but remember that even the most magical creatures come with warnings:

Allergy alert! Just like pollen causes an itchy nose, snail mucus can cause allergies in some people. Not everyone's skin likes every ingredient, which is why a skin test is your best friend. Think of it as a secret handshake; Your skin needs to be approved before you fully embrace it. Sensitive skin? Walk carefully: Sensitive skin, like a delicate shell, needs extra care.

Although snail mucus has soothing properties, it can also cause irritation in some people. Listen to your skin; Redness, itching or irritation are red flags! DIY Disaster Zone: Whispers of homemade snail slime may sound tempting but resist the urge! Sourcing ethically and ensuring good hygiene is difficult and the risks of contamination outweigh the potential benefits. Leave the science to the experts! Hidden dangers lurking:

Although most commercially available snail mucus is purified and preserved, be wary of potential contaminants such as bacteria or pesticides. deep. Choose reputable brands with transparent sourcing and processing processes. Not a panacea: Snail mucus may be the most popular, but it's not a miracle drug.

Manage your expectations and remember that consistent application of a comprehensive skin care routine is key to healthy, radiant skin. Don't give up on your other skin care heroes! Embrace the spirit of the snail: Unlocking the potential of snail mucus is more than just using a product; it's about appreciating science and respecting nature. So celebrate the natural world, make wise choices and let your skin radiate not only beauty but also ethical awareness.

After all, shining with responsibility is truly captivating and it's a beauty secret that even the cunningest fairy tale villain can't steal. Now go out, explore responsibly, and let your skin shine with the power of wise choices! Remember, knowledge is power, and when it comes to snail mucus, a little caution can go a long way. So be a savvy beauty detective, do your research and enjoy your journey to radiant skin with or without sebum!

B. Slime Squad Objective: Master the art of snail slime hunting Snail slime, the shimmering new guest to the world of skin care, promises to unleash dewy dreams and Adventure against wrinkles. But before embarking on your quest to find this slime, remove its sparkling shell and equip yourself with the knowledge to handle and preserve it like an experienced slime leader!

Remember, informed beauty shines brighter than any fairy tale spell! Picture this: a shimmering path leading to a radiant meadow, not only marking a path but also holding the potential for youthful skin. But ethical sourcing is essential, so imagine a gentle mist or playful stimulation, not a harsh extract.

Now the purified and preserved mucus awaits its journey to your face, but remember that even the most magical ingredients must be handled with care: Cleanliness is key: Think of your hands as little eggshells - they must be clean before handling mucus. Wash and disinfect thoroughly to avoid contamination, ensuring your snail slime remains a haven for healthy skin and not an unwanted guest.

Fresh and Collected: Snail mucus thrives in cool, dark environments, just as snails enjoy pink mornings. Store it in the refrigerator to preserve its potency and prevent it from turning into a science experiment gone wrong. Think of it as giving mucin a refreshing spa experience! Less is more, Slime Style: Don't go too far! A pea-sized spoonful is enough, maximising benefits without overloading your skin.

Remember that even small snails leave important traces! Patch test before peeling: Not everyone's skin likes every ingredient. Do a 24-hour patch test on the inside of your arm before applying the official snail mask. Think of it as a secret handshake; Your skin needs to be approved before you fully embrace it. Listen to your skin:

Your skin is like a wise snail, always communicating its needs. If you experience redness, itching, or irritation, take a step back. Not all snail mucus is created equal and your skin may throw a little tantrum. Ethical choices shine brightest: Choosing responsibly sourced mucus isn't just about your skin;

It's about respecting these fascinating creatures. Support brands committed to ethical practices and let your halo reflect the good choices you make. Remember, beauty with awareness truly shines! Embrace the spirit of the snail: Unlocking the potential of snail mucus is more than just using a product; it's about appreciating science and respecting nature. So celebrate the natural world, make wise choices and let your skin radiate not only beauty but also ethical awareness.

After all, shining with responsibility is truly captivating and it's a beauty secret that even the cunningest fairy tale villain can't steal. Now go out, explore responsibly, and let your skin shine with the power of wise choices! Remember, knowledge is your magic wand, and when it comes to snail mucus, just a little care can go a long way. So, be a wise beauty adventurer, follow these instructions and enjoy your journey to radiant skin, one glittering adventure at a time!

C. Stories: Search for the Term Whisperer Before Your Slime Stay Snail Mucus, the skin care world's newest shimmering guest, promises to unlock coating dreams dew and anti-wrinkle adventures. But before you embark on this dirty quest, remember: even fairy tales have wise advisors!

Consulting with a dermatologist is key to safely and effectively navigating the shimmering world of snail mucus. Think of them as a wise owl perched on a branch, guiding you through the forest with their knowledge and expertise.

Shimmering path leading to a radiant meadow, not only marking a path but also holding the potential for youthful skin. But ethical sourcing is key, so imagine a gentle mist or playful stimulation, not a harsh extract. Now purified and preserved mucus awaits its journey to your face, but remember, even the most magical ingredients can hide secrets:

Term Whisperer knows best : Don't embark on this energetic adventure alone by a snail! Dermatologists are the best skin detectives, armed with knowledge of your unique skin type, allergies, and potential sensitivities.

They will be able to decode the mysteries of snail mucus and guide you to the products that best suit your individual needs. Unravelling the mysteries of mucus: From potential allergies to interactions with other medications, a dermatologist can help you figure out the unknown.

Think of them as translators deciphering the ancient language of snail slime, ensuring a smooth, safe journey for your skin. Beyond the Hype, Real Results: Snail mucus may be trending, but dermatologists can help you separate fact from fiction.

They can evaluate the scientific evidence behind its claims and guide you toward realistic expectations, setting you up for success, not disappointment. Custom Poison and Slime Solutions: Not all snail slime is created equal! Dermatologists can recommend products formulated for your specific skin concerns, ensuring you get the most out of your snail skin care journey.

Think of them as potions masters, creating the perfect elixir just for you! Ethical choices shine brightest: Choosing responsibly sourced mucus isn't just about your skin; it's about respecting these fascinating creatures. A dermatologist can help you identify brands committed to ethical practices, allowing you to make informed choices that align with your values as beauty with awareness truly shines!

Embrace the spirit of the snail: Unlocking the potential of snail mucus is more than just using a product; it's about appreciating science and respecting nature. So celebrate the natural world, make wise choices and let your skin radiate not only beauty but also ethical awareness.

After all, shining with responsibility is truly captivating and it's a beauty secret that even the cunningest fairy tale villain can't steal. Now go out, explore responsibly and let your skin shine through the power of wise choices! Remember, your dermatologist is your trusted guide on this snail-smelling journey, so don't hesitate to seek their wisdom before diving headfirst into the unknown. After all, even the most adventurous fairy tale needs a wise advisor, and when it comes to your skin, knowledge truly is your magic medicine!

Conclusion

The Snail Story Ends: Pervasive Responsibility, Not Just Good Snail mucus, the newest glittery guest in the world of skin care, has taken us on a journey to an attractive program. We explored its potential, its complexities, and the importance of ethical sourcing and responsible use.

Remember, beauty is not just about flawless skin; it's about choices that reflect empathy and respect for the natural world. So where do you go from here? Grasp beauty trends with knowledge: Don't blindly follow trends.

Always be curious, research and choose products that align with your values. Remember, knowledge is power and when it comes to your skin, it is your ultimate shield. Let your choices shine:

Support brands committed to ethical sourcing and sustainable practices. Your light reflects not only the magic of snail mucus but also the responsibility you demonstrate. Celebrate the natural world: Snail mucus is a gift from nature, so cherish its wonders.

Explore other natural ingredients, learn about their origins, and enjoy the magic that lurks beneath the surface. Listen to your skin. Your skin is your wisest advisor. Pay attention to their needs, experiment thoughtfully, and find what works best for you. Remember, beauty is a journey, not a destination, so enjoy the exploration! And finally,

Remember this: true beauty shines from within. It's about confidence, self-love and the choices you make, not just the products you use. Embrace your unique journey, celebrate your individuality, and let your inner light shine. After all, the most seductive brilliance comes from being true to yourself. So go forth, explore and shine! The world needs your unique, savvy, responsible and incredibly outstanding beauty brand.

A. Shell Yes, but do it right: Ethical Snail Mucus Extract Summary Snail mucus, the shimmering new guest of the skin care world, has caught the attention of We promise rosy dreams and anti-wrinkle adventures. But before we start this sleazy hunting trip, let's take a step back and focus on the most important aspect:

ethical and responsible mining of even fairy tales have heroes who fight for the good guys, and in this case, the good guys are the snails! Picture this: a shimmering path leading to a glowing meadow, but instead of marking a path, it symbolises the journey of the mucus itself.

We want this journey to be filled with gentle and playful stimulation, not harsh extractive actions that harm these fascinating creatures. Ethical sourcing is more than just a buzzword; it is the foundation of true beauty. So why is proper extraction so important? Snail Serenity: Imagine the tiny snails being stressed and uncomfortable during the extraction process.

Not only is it heartbreaking, but it can also affect the quality of mucus. We want snails to be happy, gliding through their days, happily leaving behind their slimy, magical trail. Sustainability Issues: Responsible agricultural practices ensure healthy snail populations and sustainable mucus sources for generations to come. Think of it as caring for a fragile ecosystem where both snails and humans can thrive.

Purity Matters: Harsh extraction methods can introduce contaminants like bacteria or pesticides, potentially harming your skin instead of improving it. We want pure, ethically sourced mucus, like a sparkling stream from a wholesome source.
Respect Matters: These sleazy friends deserve our respect. By choosing brands that are committed to ethical practices, we show the world that beauty should not come at the expense of the well-being of others.

Remember that true beauty shines through responsibility. Don't let the allure of snail mucus blind you to the importance of ethical sourcing. Choose brands that prioritise the health of snails, the environment and ultimately your own skin. So next time you use a snail slime product, remember this: shine bright, but shine responsibly.

Let your light reflect your wise choices and your empathy for the natural world. Together, we can create a beautiful story where everyone wins, people, snails and the planet itself. Now go ahead, explore ethically and let your skin sparkle with the power of responsible choices!

B. Indulge yourself in slime goodness: Discover the snail's path to radiant skin Snail mucus, the skin care world's newest sticky muse, sounds like a fairy potion, but hold on to your glass slippers! This gooey treasure holds the potential for rosy dreams and wrinkle-defying adventures,

if you approach it with curiosity and make responsible choices. Imagine this: child architects leave behind trails of glitter that not only mark their path but also offer the key to radiant skin. Ethical sourcing is paramount, so consider gentle misting rather than harsh extraction.

Now, with the mucus safely collected, the magic is waiting for you to discover: Hydration Harmony: Imagine a dry desert transformed into a lush oasis. Uh Snail mucus, rich in hyaluronic acid, can help your skin retain moisture, leaving it plump and dewy - just like a snail gliding through the morning dew.

Anti-wrinkle waltz: Will wrinkles fade away? Yes, please! Snail mucus contains peptides and other benefits that can help stimulate collagen production, resulting in smoother, more youthful skin. Imagine the lines on your face softening like the ripples of a still lake.

Gentle Serenade: Sensitive skin? Snail mucus could be your new best friend! Its anti-inflammatory properties can help soothe redness and irritation, leaving your skin like a peaceful meadow after a light rain.

ḤBrightening Bonanza: Boring no more! Snail mucus can help gently exfoliate and brighten your skin, revealing skin that glows as brightly as the first rays of sunlight after a storm. But remember, the journey is important: Ethical exploration:

Choose brands committed to responsible snail farming and harvesting practices. Support happy snails, happy skin and a happy planet! Slow start: Don't dive headfirst into a puddle of slime! Test a patch and gradually introduce mucus to see how your skin reacts. Think of it as a cautious snail exploring its new territory.

Visit Skincare Sage: Not sure? Ask your dermatologist for advice. They can assess your needs and recommend the best treatment for your unique skin. Embrace the spirit of the snail: Unlocking the potential of snail mucus is more than just using a product; it's about appreciating science and respecting nature.

Celebrate the natural world, make wise choices and let your skin radiate not only beauty but also ethical awareness. So, are you ready to embark on this unique skin care adventure? Remember, the most captivating brilliance comes from exploring responsibly and embracing the magic that lies in the unexpected. So don't be afraid to get a little slimy: your bright future could be waiting for you on the slimy trail of a snail!

C .Yeah, You Can Shine Responsibly: Final Thoughts on Snail Mucus Odyssey The journey through the glittering world of snail slime is fascinating. We've explored its potential benefits, dug deeper into ethical sourcing and revealed the importance of responsible choices. But before we end the book with this fascinating chapter, let's leave you with some final thoughts and recommendations:

Remember that you are not Cinderella and this is not a magic potion of the fairy godmother. Snail mucus may have promise but it is not a miracle cure. Consistent use of a comprehensive skin care routine tailored to your unique needs is essential to achieving and maintaining radiant skin. Think of it as building a beautiful garden where many different elements work together to achieve optimal growth.

Embrace the spirit of the snail: Slow, steady progress and respect for nature. Don't rush through this process or expect results overnight. Give your skin time to adjust and appreciate the natural world that gives us this fascinating ingredient. Let it be a lesson in the snail's patient journey, leaving behind a trail of sparkling beauty.

Be an informed explorer, not a blind follower of trends. Do your research, ask questions and choose brands that are committed to transparency, ethical sourcing and sustainable practices. Your wise choices can make a difference, not only for your skin but also for the well-being of these tiny architects and the planet they inhabit. Remember, true beauty shines from within and that includes the choices you make.

Don't be afraid to experiment, but always start cautiously. Do a patch test, listen to your skin, and consult a dermatologist if necessary. Remember that your skin is unique and what works for someone else may not work for you. Be your own skin care detective and find out what makes your skin tick!

Finally, remember that the most seductive light is the light that comes from being true to yourself. Embrace your individuality, celebrate your unique beauty, and let your inner light shine. After all, confidence and self-love are the most powerful beauty elixirs you can find. So, as you finish this chapter on snail mucus, remember this: you have the power to choose, to explore, and to exercise responsibility. Go ahead and live your own unique skin care journey, one wise decision and one streak of sparkle at a time!